Hi Everyone !!! Welcome to my Little Smoothie Book !!!

Please remember that this is a guide – yes, some of the smoothies here are particularly scrumptious, but you don't have to make every smoothie exactly how I do! We eat everything fresh. The only fruits that I use frozen (usually) are berries, coconut, sometimes pineapple, rarely anything else. I prefer using a little ice, and a little water as my liquid. I have yet to experience a watered down smoothie !! The trick is not to add too much water – we like our smoothies on the thick side and my husband likes his chilled, hence the ice (just a little ice). If you add a little more ice, you will get a slushie, which can be delicious as well !!! You do not have to add ice and/or water – that is totally up to you. I'm sharing with you how I make my smoothies and how we enjoy them. Not every single smoothie needs liquid added to it. Make your smoothies how YOU like them !!! Remember, you can always add ingredients, but once you put them in, you can't remove them !!!

Most of the smoothies here are 32oz – a great way to start the day !!!

If you like your smoothies a little sweeter, then add a little stevia or whatever your favorite sweetener is. I sometimes put a few drops of stevia in my smoothies just to take away any bitterness that some of the not-so-sweet fruits may impart. That's just fine!! Please do what makes you happy!

Many fruits with skin should be peeled, such as bananas, lemons, mango, papaya, kiwi – use your discretion. I use a Blendtec high speed blender to make my smoothies. You may not achieve smoothness if you do not use a high speed blender such as a Blendtec or Vitamix. If that's OK with you, then it's perfect!

You may not be able to get some of the fruits I use, and that's OK too. Leave them out – you will still have a delicious smoothie! This is not an exact science.

I look forward to seeing you on my website, rawchefjane.com, and on my Facebook page, RAW CHEF JANE and on Instagram, rawchefjane. Remember It's Not Just Salad and Jane's Daily Thoughts are both available on Amazon as well !!!

I encourage you to use your creativity!! And, remember to always make your smoothie with love and drink it with gratitude!   Enjoy!!! Love and Blessings always to everyone . . .

RCJ

1. Smoothie for two today:

2 Bananas
1 lemon
1/2 Cup Papaya
1/2 Cup Raspberries

Put all ingredients into your high speed blender, add a little ice and a little water. Enjoy.

2. Smoothie for One:

1 Banana
1 Mango
1 Lemon
1/4 Cup Blackberries

Place ingredients into your blender, add ice and water if desired. Blend it up and enjoy!

3. RAW CHEF JANE's SMOOTHIE for TWO

1 Banana
1 Peach
1 Lemon
1 Apple
¼ Cup Raspberries
¼ Cup Blackberries
½ Cup Strawberries
¼ Cup Pineapple

Place everything into your high speed blender. Add ice and/or water as desired. Blend and enjoy!

4. Creamsicle Smoothie for One:

1 large orange
1 large banana
A little ice

This is a really simple smoothie and really delicious !!!

Blend. Drink. Enjoy.

5. Green Smoothie:

1 Banana
1 Mango
1 Lemon
1 Kiwi
Some Strawberries

2 Cups spinach (that's what I was able to pick from the garden this morning)

Blend, adding ice and water if desired. Way Yum.

6. Cherry Chocolate Smoothie:

20 Pitted Cherries
2 Small Bananas
2 TBS Raw Cacao Powder
Stevia for desired sweetness
Ice

Blend. Drink. Enjoy.

7. Very Berry Smoothie

1 Banana
¼ Cup Blackberries
¼ Cup Raspberries
4 LARGE Strawberries or about 1 cup or so
1 Kiwi
Ice, as desired
Water if needed – add just a little at a time if you need to

Peel Banana and Kiwi. Add all ingredients to blender, adding ice
and/or water as desired. Blend it up and enjoy !

8. Tropical Smoothie for Two:

2 Bananas
1-2 Cups Strawberries
1 Lemon
1 Kiwi
¾ Cup Papaya
¾ Cup Pineapple
Ice, as desired
A little water, if needed

Peel Bananas, Kiwi and Lemon. Hull Strawberries. Add all
ingredients to Blender, blend and enjoy.

9. Nice Big Smoothie for the day:

1 Banana
2 Apricots
1 Apple
1 Lemon
small piece of fresh ginger

Blend it up, adding ice and water as desired.

10. 32 oz Smoothie of the day:

½ Cup Coconut (I use the frozen, without any additives)
½ Cup Pineapple
1 Orange
1 Lemon
1 Banana

Blend and enjoy. Make it and drink it with love and gratitude !!!

11. Delicious Tropical Smoothie:

1 Banana
¼ Cup Raspberries
1 Kiwi
½ Lemon
2 Small Peaches
A little Ice and a little water as desired

Blend it up as you like it and enjoy !!!

12. Today's Amazing Smoothie for Two:

2 Bananas
1 Kiwi
1 Lemon
½ Cup Pineapple
½ Cup Blackberries
8-10 Large Strawberries
Ice as desired
A little water if needed

This is our favorite smoothie!!! It's really good.

13. Smoothie for today:

I banana
1 mango
½ lemon
2 small peaches
1 very generous cup of strawberries

Ice and water as desired. Blend it up !!!

14. Today's Smoothie for Two:

2 Bananas
1 Mango
1 Lemon
1 Cup Papaya
½ Cup Raspberries

Way Yum !!!

15. Simple Summer Smoothie

1 Banana
2-2 ½ Cups Strawberries
1 Kiwi

Blend and Enjoy !!!

16. Richard's Smoothie

4 Apricots
1 Kiwi
1 Lemon
1 Mango
½ Cup Raspberries

Blend it up adding ice, water and sweetener as desired!

17. Large Smoothie for One Today

3 Small Peaches
1 Kiwi
2 Cups Strawberries
Ice/water as desired

Blend and enjoy!

18. Today's Smoothie for two:

2 Bananas
10 Cherries (pitted)
1 Kiwi
1 Apple
¾ Cup Pineapple
1 Mango
Ice/Water as desired

Blend it up and enjoy, adding ice and water if desired !!!

19. Simple and Delicious Smoothie

1 Banana
1 Mango
1 Lemon
½ Cup Raspberries

Water and Ice as desired. One of my favorites !!!

20. Monday Morning Smoothie

1 Cup Fresh Spinach
1 Banana
1 Lemon
1 Kiwi
¼ - ½ Cup Raspberries
¼ - ½ Cup Blackberries

Ice and water as desired. Blend and enjoy.

21. The Way Yum Smoothie

1 Banana
1 Kiwi
1 Lemon
1 Cup Strawberries
½ Cup Pineapple
1 Guava

Ice/Water as desired. Blend and Enjoy!

22. Big Smoothie of the Day

2 Apricots (pitted)
½ Dragon Fruit
1 Mango
1 Cup Blackberries
1 Kiwi
1 Plum (pitted)

Ice and water as desired. Blend and Enjoy

23. First Day of Summer Smoothie

1 Banana
1 Lemon
1 Guava
1 Cup Blueberries
5 Strawberries
¼ Cup Blackberries
1 Peach

Ice and water as desired. Blend it up !!!

24. Second Day of Summer Smoothie

1 Banana
1 Guava
1 Lemon
½ Cup Coconut
¼ Cup Pineapple
¼ Cup Blackberries
¼ Cup Raspberries
1 Kiwi

Ice and Water as desired. Blend and enjoy…This is a good one!!!

25. Tropical Summer Smoothie

Two Mangoes
4 Peaches
1 Lemon
½ Cup Raspberries

You know what to do !!! Perfect Tropical Summer Smoothie !!

26. Most Excellent Summer Smoothie for Two

1 Mango
2 Peaches
1 Guava
1 Lemon
1 Kiwi
1 Cup Blueberries
1 Cup Blackberries

Ice and water as desired. Blend it up and enjoy !

27. Peaches are in Season Smoothie !

6 Small Peaches
1 Banana
1 Lemon
1 Mango

Blend it up with some ice and water, as desired !

28. Another Summer Smoothie

1 Apple
1 Lemon
1 Kiwi
½ Cup Pineapple
4 Peaches

Add a little ice and a little water, blend it up and enjoy!!!

29. Summer Smoothie for One

1 Banana
1 Lemon
1Guava
3 Peaches
½ Cup Raspberries

Ice and water as desired . . . blend and enjoy!

30. The Holy Cow this is Delicious Smoothie

1-2 Bananas
1 Kiwi
6 Strawberries
1 Lemon
½ Cup Raspberries
½ Cup Blackberries
3 Peaches

Blend it up and enjoy !!!

31. Supreme Sunday Summer Smoothie

1 Cup Papaya
1 Cup Strawberries
1 Mango
1 Lemon
1 Kiwi
3 Peaches

Ice and Water as desired . . . you know what to do !!!

32. Summer Holiday Smoothie

1 Banana
1 Guava
1 Lemon
1 Cup Papaya
½ Cup Strawberries
½ Cup Raspberries
½ Cup Blackberries

Makes a nice big smoothie !!! Blend it up with ice/water to your
liking. Enjoy!

33. Tuesday Morning Smoothie

2 Bananas
1 Mango
½ Dragon Fruit
1 Lemon
1 Kiwi
1 Cup Strawberries

Ice and water as desired. YUM.

34. Saturday Smoothie

1 Banana
1 Lemon
1 Mango
1 Guava
3 Peaches
1 Cup Strawberries

Add Ice and water as desired. I find that a cup of ice usually does the trick. Blend it up and enjoy !!!

35. Simple Sunday Smoothie

1 Cup Papaya
1 Cup Strawberries
2 Kiwis

Ice and a little water as desired. Blend it up. This one has a wow factor !!!

36. Monday Morning Wake Up Smoothie

2 Apricots
2 Peaches
1 Mango
1 Banana
1 Lemon
1/3 Cup Raspberries

Add all ingredients to your Blender and enjoy. Way Yumilicious!!!!!

37. Tuesday Smeusday

1 Cup Papaya
1 Cup Blackberries
1 Guava
1 Mango

Ice. Water. Blend.

38. Wonderful Wednesday Smoothie

1 Banana
6 Peaches
¼ Cup Raspberries

Blend it up with a little ice and a little water !!!

39. Thursday Smoothie

1 Banana
1 Lemon
1/3 Cup Blackberries
1 Apple
1 Guava
1 Kiwi

Add a little ice and a little water . . . blend and enjoy !!!

40. Friday Freshness

1 Banana
1 Lemon
12 Cherries (pitted of course)
1 Mango

Simple one today, and really delicious !!

41. Monday Morning Eye Opener Smoothie

1 Large Banana
2 Cups Strawberries
2 Kiwis

Add some ice and blend. I didn't add water to this one, but do
what makes you happy !!!

42. Wonderful Wednesday Smoothie

2 Large Bananas or 3 Small Bananas
2 Lemons
1 Cup Raspberries

Ice, A Little Water, Blend, Enjoy !!

43. Thursday Morning Smoothie

2 Bananas
4 Peaches
½ Cup Raspberries
1 small piece of fresh ginger

Add a little ice and water and blend it up !!!

44. Friday Smoothie for Two

1 Lime
1 Cup Coconut
2 Cups Blueberries
1-2 Bananas

Add a little ice and a little water and enjoy !

45. Hot Summer Day Smoothie

1-2 Bananas
1 Kiwi
1 Cup Strawberries
1 Lemon
1 Cup Blueberries

Add a little ice and a little water, then blend !!

46. Sunday Summer Smoothie

1 Lemon
2 Cups Blueberries
1 Banana
1 Piece of Ginger

Add some ice and water as desired . . . YUM !!!

47. Monday Smoothie for One

1 Lemon
1 Kiwi
1 Cup Blueberries
1 Peach
1 Banana
1 Piece of Ginger

Add a little ice. Add a little water. Blend it up !!!

48. Tuesday's Tasty Smoothie

2 Lemons
½ Cup Raspberries
5 Peaches
1 Piece of Ginger
1 Banana

Add a little ice, a little water, blend and enjoy !!!

49. A Thursday Smoothie for Two

2 Kiwis
2 Bananas
2 Cups Blueberries
½ Cup Raspberries
1 Piece of Ginger

A little ice, a little water, blend it up!

50. Spectacular Saturday Smoothie

1 Lemon
½ Cup Dragon Fruit
½ Cup Blackberries
½ Cup Raspberries
1 Piece of Ginger
1 Banana
½ Mango

Blend it up with a little ice and a little water !!!

51. Lazy Sunday Smoothie

1 Lemon
1 Kiwi
1 Banana
1 Apple
½ Mango
Piece of Ginger

Add a little ice and a little water, blend and enjoy !

52. Monday Moothie

1 Lemon
1 Kiwi
1 Cup Blueberries
1 Banana
1 Piece of Ginger
½ Cup Dragon Fruit

Add a little ice and water as desired, then blend it up !!!

53. Twosday Smoothie for Two

2 Lemons
2 Bananas
1 Cup Blueberries
1 Cup Raspberries
1 Piece of Ginger
1 Mango

Add a little ice and a tiny bit of water if you'd like, blend it up and enjoy !

54. Wild Wednesday Smoothie

1 Mango
2 Apriums
1 Cup Raspberries
1 Banana
½ Cup Pineapple
1 Piece of Ginger

Add a little Ice and a little water, blend and love it !!

55. Smoothie for a Rainy Saturday

4 Peaches
1 Lemon
1 Guava
1 Mango
1 Cup Papaya
1 Piece of Ginger

Add a little ice, blend it up and enjoy! Way Yum !!

56. Six Peach Sunday Smoothie

6 Peaches (I like to cut my peaches in half, take out the pit, and
scrape out the insides without the skin, as I'm very allergic to the
skin)
1 Piece of Ginger
1 Cup of Ice

Blend it. It comes out amazingly creamy and luscious !

57. Four Peaches and a Banana Smoothie

4 Peaches
1 Banana
1 Lemon
1 Piece of Ginger

Add a little Ice, Blend it up and enjoy!

58. Grapey Smoothie

2 Cups Concord Grapes
1 ½ Cups Pineapple
2 Lemons

Add some ice and you may need a little stevia in this one. Blend it up and enjoy !!!

59. Peach/Blackberry/Guava Smoothie

4 Peaches
2 Cups Blackberries
1 Guava

Add a little ice, blend and enjoy!!!

60. Rainy Day Smoothie for Two

2 Bananas
1 Mango
1 Cup Papaya
1 Lemon
1 Peach
1 Cup Raspberries
1 Cup Blackberries
1 Piece of Ginger
1 Guava

What's in YOUR Blender?

61. Awakening Smoothie

3 Peaches
1 Cup Raspberries
1 Cup Blackberries
½ Lemon
1 Guava
1 Banana
1 Cup Papaya

What a flavor this one has !!! What's in your Blender?

62. Raspberry/Peach Smoothie

5 Peaches
2 Cups Raspberries
Small piece of ginger (optional)

WAYYYYYYY YUM !!!!!! What's in YOUR Blender?

63. The Way Good Smoothie

1 Kiwi
1 Guava
1 Cup Papaya
1 Banana
½ of a Dragon Fruit
1 Pluot

Blend it up with a little ice (If desired) and a little water . . . What's
in YOUR Blender?

64. Wonderful Wednesday Smoothie

1 Lemon
1 Guava
1 Apple
1 Banana
1 Cup Raspberries

Add a little ice & water, blend it up and enjoy !

65. Thirsty Thursday Smoothie

1 Kiwi
1 Lemon
1 Peach
1 Banana
1 Apple
1 Mango
1 Small Piece of Ginger (always optional)

Blend with a little ice and water, if desired. Way YUMMM !!!!

66. Foggy Tuesday Morning Smoothie

2 Nectarines
1 Peach
½ Mango
1 Lemon

Add a little ice and a little water, blend it up !!! What's in YOUR Smoothie?

67. Sunny Wednesday Morning Smoothie

1 Lemon
1 Nectarine
2 Peaches
2 Plumcots

A little ice. A little water. What's in YOUR Smoothie ???

68. Cloudy Thursday Smoothie for Two

1 Banana
1 Lemon
1 Kiwi
1 Guava
1 Nectarine
2 Peaches
½ Mango
½ Cup Raspberries
½ Cup Blackberries
1 small piece of Ginger

Add some ice and water, blend it up and enjoy!!

69. Foggy Friday Smoothie

1 Banana
1 Apple
2 Key Limes
½ of a Dragon Fruit
1 Peach
¼ Cup Raspberries

Add a little ice and a little water and enjoy !!! What's in YOUR
Blender?

70. Sunny Saturday Smoothie

1 Apple
1 Peach
2 Bananas
½ Cup Blackberries
½ Cup Blueberries
1 Piece of Ginger
1 Lemon

Add some ice. Add a little water. Blend it up and get healthy !!!
What's in YOUR Blender?

71. Birthday Smoothie

3 Bananas
2 Lemons
½ Cup Raspberries

Add a little ice and a little water, blend it up and be prepared for a
wow moment !!! What's in YOUR Smoothie ???

72. Day After My Birthday Smoothie

1 Lemon
3 Bananas
5 Figs
¼ Cup Blackberries

Add a little Ice and water, blend and enjoy !!

73. Tuesday Smoosday

1 Banana
1 Lemon
1 Guava
1 Apple
1 Cup Blueberries

Add a little ice and water as needed. Blend it up and enjoy!
What's in your Blender?

74. Smoothie for a Wednesday Morning

2 Lemons
½ Cup Honeydew
1 Cup Cantaloupe
½ Cup Grapes
1 Banana
½ Cup Watermelon

Add a little ice and blend it up !!! What's in YOUR Blender?

75. Sunny Friday Smoothie

2 Lemons
2 Guavas
2 Bananas
1 Kiwi
½ Cup Raspberries

Add a little ice and water, blend it up and nourish your body !!

76. Sunny Sunday Smoothie

1 Lemon
1 Mango
1 Banana
2 Cups Blueberries

Add some ice and water, blend it up and enjoy !!

77. First Day of Fall Smoothie

1-2 Bananas
1 Heaping Cup of Strawberries (about 14)
1 Kiwi

Add a little ice and water as desired, blend it up !!!

78. Fall Friday Smoothie

1 Lemon
1 Kiwi
½ of a Mango
½ Cup Raspberries
1 Banana

Add a little Ice and water as desired, blend and enjoy !

79. Cloudy Saturday Smoothie

1-2 Bananas
1 Cup Papaya
1 Lemon
1 Cup Strawberries

Add a little ice and blend it up !!!

Sunny Munday Smoothie

1 Lemon
2 Kiwis
1 Banana
½ of a Mango
½ Cup Papaya
¼ Cup Blackberries

Add a little ice and water if desired, blend it up and enjoy !!!

80. Last Day of September Smoothie

1 Lemon
1 Mango
1 Cup Papaya
1 Kiwi
1 Banana
½ Cup Raspberries

Add a little ice and water as desired, blend it up and enjoy !

81. Moody Monday Smoothie

1 Lemon
1 Mango
¼ Cup Pomegranate Seeds
2 Bananas

Add a little ice and water as desired . . . blend it up !!!!

82. Fall Tuesday Smoothie

2 Bananas
2 Lemons
½ Cup Raspberries

Add a little ice, if desired and blend it up !!

83. A Wednesday Smoothie

2 Cups Papaya
1 Lemon
½ Cup Pomegranate
1 Banana

Add a little ice and water as desired !!!

84. Saturday Afternoon Smoothie

1 Banana
1 Mango
2 TBS Pomegranate
1 Lemon
2 Figs

Add a little ice and water as desired !! Blend it up and enjoy !

85. Smoothie for a Fall Morning

1 Kiwi
1 Lemon
1 Banana
1 Cup Papaya

Blend it up with a little ice (as desired) and a little water !

86. Frosty Friday Smoothie

1 Lemon
1 Apple
1 Banana
½ - 1 Cup Papaya

Add a little water and ice as desired. Blend and enjoy !

87. Fall Saturday Smoothie

1 Banana
1 Lemon
1 Kiwi
½ - ¾ Cup Raspberries

Add a little ice (if desired) and water – blend it up !!

88. Moody Monday Smoothie

1 Lemon
½ Cup Blueberries
¼ Cup Blackberries
1 Banana
1½ Pear (or just 1 or 2)
4-6 Figs

Add a little ice and water as desired. Blend and Enjoy !!

89. Fall Sunday Morning Smoothie

1 Kiwi
½ Cup Raspberries
5 Figs
½ Cup Pineapple
1 Banana

Ice and water as desired. Blend it up !!!

90. Halloween Smoothie

1 Lemon
6 Figs
1 Pear
1 Banana

Add a little ice and water as desired, blend it up and enjoy !!!

91. Special Sunday Smoothie

1 Kiwi
1 Guava
1 Banana
½-3/4 Cup of Cranberries

Add some ice and a little water as desired. Blend and enjoy !!!

92. Fall Thursday Smoothie

½ Cup Cranberries
1 Pear
1 Lemon
1 Banana

If you'd like to add some ice and water, then do ! Blend and enjoy!

93. Snow on the Mountain Smoothie

1 Persimmon
3-4 chunks of Pineapple or 1 Lemon
1 Banana
½ Cup Cranberries
1 Guava

Add a little ice and water as desired. Blend it up and enjoy !!

94. Chilly Morning Smoothie

½ Banana
1 Lemon
1 Cup Cranberries
1 Small Apple

Add some ice and water as desired. Blend and enjoy !!!

95. Smoothie for a Very Cold Thursday

½ Cup Cranberries
1/3 Cup Pomegranate Seeds
½ Banana
1 Lemon
1 Guava
½ Persimmon

Add ice and water as desired. Blend it up and enjoy !!!

96. Tastes Like Candy on a Sunday Morning Smoothie

½ Banana
1 Apple
1 Pear
1 Lemon
¾ Cup Cranberries

Blend it up and enjoy !!! Add a little water and ice as desired !

97. Sunny Monday Smoothie

1 Lemon
¾ Cup Cranberries
1 Guava
½ Persimmon
½ Banana

Add a little ice and water if desired, blend it up and enjoy !!!

98. Thankful Thursday Smoothie

1 Lemon
½ Cup Pomegranate
2 Guavas
½ Banana
1 Small Apple

Add a little ice and water as desired. Blend and Enjoy !!!

99. Good Ole' Green Smoothie

1 Banana
½ Cup Cranberries
1 Lemon
1 Small Apple
2 Cups Spinach

Add a little water and ice as desired, then blend it up !!!

100. Monday Morning Moothie

1 Guava
1 Banana
1 Lemon
2-3 Cups Spinach

Add a little ice and water as desired, blend it up and enjoy !!!

101. Cloudy Rainy Tuesday Smoosday

1 Lemon
½ Mango
1/3 Cup Cranberries
1/3 Cup Raspberries
1 Banana
1 Pear

Add a little water and ice if desired. Blend and get fit and healthy !!!

102. December Morning Smoothie

2 Kiwis
1 Lemon
1 Guava
½ Cup Raspberries
1 Banana
½ Mango

Add water and ice as desired. Blend and enjoy -- this is a really good one !!!

103. Sunny Saturday Smoothie

1 Lemon
1 Kiwi
½ Cup Blueberries
½ Cup Cranberries
1 Banana
1 Guava

Add a little ice and water if desired, blend and enjoy !!!

104. Almost Winter Wednesday Smoothie

1 Guava
1 Kiwi
1 Banana
1 Apple
1 Lemon
½ Cup Pomegranate
¼ Cup Raspberries

Add some ice and water as desired, blend and be grateful !!!

105. New Year's Eve Smoothie

1 Banana
1 Kiwi
1/3 Cup Pineapple
½ Cup Raspberries

Add ice and water if desired, blend it up and live in love!!!

106. Tuesday Smoosday

½ Mango
½ Banana
1 Lemon
1 Apple
¼ Cup Pineapple
¼ Cup Cranberries

Add some water and ice as desired, blend and enjoy !